Nine Lives and Still Running

Nine Lives and Still Running

By Tony Perez

iUniverse, Inc.

New York Lincoln Shanghai

Nine Lives and Still Running

iUniverse, Inc.

For information address:
iUniverse, Inc.
2021 Pine Lake Road, Suite 100
Lincoln, NE 68512
www.iuniverse.com

ISBN: 0-595-32303-0

Printed in the United States of America

Contents

Acknowledgements

"Whoever saves one life saves the world entirely." When I meditate upon this inspiring quote from the Hebrew Talmud, I am emphatically grateful for those friends God has placed in my path. After approximately seven years of battling brain cancer, chemo-therapy, radiation, and other challenges, I am deeply indebted to friends. I want to thank those people for their prayers, support, and counseling; who unselfishly went beyond the call to see God miraculously intervene during those trying times. Furthermore, it is with great conviction that I declare it is solely God's Grace that has sustained me to put this testimony in print. I dedicate it to the sacred memory of the countless victims and their families whose battle with this deadly disease was to no avail. May the peace of God be with you.

To begin with, I want to thank my lovely and precious wife, Carol, who day and night, regardless of my predictable situation stood by my bedside despite staring death in the face time after time. Her support as a Minister of the Gospel kept me (and still keeps me) strong in my faith through that particular ordeal and more. Together we have determined to face the future and press on. To my mother Beatriz Sosa, I am grateful for all her prayers and for being a woman of God. Thank you for your guidance and for always being that wonderful mother to me. Currently, I am a student with a double major in Special Education and Nursing at the University of Texas Pan-American.

To Pastor Hector and Alma Rodriguez: Thank you for your friendship and support. Without it the way would not have been paved to write this book. To the late Rev. Ron Bowen, whom I knew as a man of prayer and has gone to be with the Lord, thank you for the opportunity to sit and learn under your leadership. Also, I want to thank you Bud and Esther Weisman for your help in my recovery during my physical therapy. Rev. Greg Thurstenson, Gracias for the generosity and courtesy you showed driving me to and from M. D. Anderson during my chemotherapy treatments. Mr. and Mrs. Bill Fickling, thank you for graciously opening your home and hearts to me, I give special thanks. To Alex Sanders, thank you for showing me Jesus through your example, and not just your words. Furthermore, special thanks are in order for you Mr. and Mrs. Clark Spike for your generosity during my treatments. Mr. and Mrs. Jim and Linda

Deckock, thank you for your unconditional support. To my family members: thank you for your prayers, support, and help. Last but not least, thank you Rebecca Bontrager for spending countless numbers of hours revising, editing, and giving me the general help in putting my story together. Thank you for your servant hood and friendship. In Belfast, Northern Ireland, thank you to those at CFC Church. In Clang, Malaysia, thank you to those at Glad Tidings Assembly of God. To my medical doctors, especially Dr. Curtis Maynard, thank you for your friendship and encouragement during my recovery and regular visits. In addition, Dr. Reymond Sawaya, Dr. Alfred Yung, and Gloria Humphry, R.N. at M.D. Anderson Cancer Center.

Foreword

What comes to mind when we say names like Noah or Enoch or Lydia? Most of us know these names as people from the Old or New Testaments. We know them because of their wonderful and sometimes miraculous stories. How exciting to think of young David, son of Jesse standing against that giant Goliath. How thrilling to imagine Gideon blowing the trumpet and defeating the Midianites. And who wouldn't want to be standing there next to Mary Magdalene as she told the disciples that Jesus had actually risen from the dead!

The Bible is filled with wonderful stories about real people. And although the Bible is complete, the list of stories of real people experiencing the wonderful miracles of God is not. Real miracles still happen to real people today; and Tony Perez is one of those miracle people. Now, miracles do not happen because we somehow win God's favor by being especially good or holy. It is an unfortunate truth that many Godly people have not experienced the physical miracle of healing, only to realize the spiritual miracle of eternal life. No, miracles happen because they fit into God's plan for the life of a person. He and He alone knows what is best for each of us who seek after Him. God chose to touch the life and body of Tony. And, amazingly enough, He did not choose to do it just once, but many times. He chooses to keep Tony here on earth with us for another season to encourage us, to challenge us, and to inspire us to keep our eyes always on Jesus.

You may not know Tony personally, but I can tell you that he is a man like Noah and King David and Gideon. He is a man who wants to live his life to the glory of God. You will find by reading this book that, as Tony chose to keep his eyes on Jesus through his challenging ordeal of life, God was able to speak to him and encourage him. You too will be blessed, as I was, as God speaks to you through *Nine Lives and Still Running*—Tony's exciting modern day miracle.

Bruce A. Sonnenberg
He Intends Victory
The Village Church of Irvine
5 Wrigley
Irvine, CA 92618

Preface

*"But when she could no longer hide him (Moses), she took an ark of bul-
rushes for him, daubed it with asphalt and pitch, put the child in it, and
laid it in the river's bank."*

—Exodus 2:3

A cruel pharaoh attempts to wipe out the Jewish race by killing all the male chil-
dren—but Moses escapes, hidden in the bulrushes, the future deliverer of his
people.

Herod, hearing of a threat to his throne, decrees a massacre of all male babies
under two years of age—but Joseph is warned by an angel, and Jesus is whisked
away to Egypt until it's safe for Him to return.

The tactics of Satan haven't changed much in 4,000 years. He is still trying to
steal, kill and destroy. He desperately wants to destroy the lives of potential
world-changers; that is, anyone who might one day sell out totally in devotion
and service to Jesus Christ. In other words—YOU!

Even as the blood of 5,000 aborted babies per day in America cries out, I stand
in awe and gratitude at the hedge of protection that God has placed around my
life. It has not been fate; it has not been coincidence. As you read my story, I pray
that you will be encouraged to trust the wisdom of God no matter what trials and
tribulations He may allow into your life.

HALLELUJAH! HE IS IN CONTROL!

Introduction

We were in the process of starting a revolution. I asked everyone to close their eyes, bow their heads and pray along with me out loud. Standing in a circle holding hands, I felt my whole body shaking in fear not knowing for certain if what we were doing was "legal" or not. At the center of the school grounds, in front of the library, and in view of the main office, we stood as modern day radicals to express our newfound convictions. In efforts to quiet down my conscious anxiety, I asked everyone to pray louder as they followed my lead. With my eyes tightly shut as to try to repel fear from the already developing crowd around us, I began to speak in tongues. In the distance I could hear people murmuring their thoughts about the visible commotion presented by us. I peeked open my left eye, hoping no one was watching and that the crowd would soon fade away, but as I did, in the distance, I caught the eyes of the local school principal that stood watching. His face had a look of disdained and disapproval. Instantly, my fear turns to exhilarating joy…I now knew our cause was on the way to provoke a wave of change. This was the instigation of our visible revolution to proclaiming our faith.

This led us to begin a weekly Bible study in a local high school campus. Our meetings brought in youth from all walks of like. In a sense to defy the infamous Church vs. State decision, our club was anything but ordinary. In fact, we were the cause of many debates. This caused the local school district Superintendent to get involved. His decision was to allow us to keep on meeting in the local high school grounds as long as we kept all the rules and regulations required of all school clubs.

It was during one of our meetings that I was introduced to an athletic runner that came from the "other side of the tracks". He was invited to come and visit these radical Christians who met every Thursday morning in Room G-19 to express their faith in Christ. Like many, he came to "check it out" to see what these crazy kids were doing. Fortunately, God h ad other plans for him and for the other that "dropped" by out of curiosity. Most left changed because of what Christ did in their lives.

Tony was a member of the track team and a superb long distance runner. His life revolved around being the best on the field. He felt alive when he participated in track events; they were his dream, his passion, and his life's goal. Winning events were his ticket out of poverty and the new road towards scholarships and education. Many school scouts were sent to interview his athletic ability; many liked what they saw. They offered great dreams, good college grants, and a great opportunity to become part of leading university track teams.

It was during this time that Tony's life began to change. He approached me one day and asked me about discipleship. As our friendship continued to develop, we came up with a resolution. Every Thursday, during lunch time, we were to meet under the tree by the tennis courts for one-on-one discipleship. And so it was; for a whole year, Tony and I studied, prayed, and read the scriptures during the hot Texas heat under the tree in the middle of the school yard. It was here that our lives took a shift in our walk with Christ.

Under the tree God began a work in us both and friendship that has succeeded crisis, struggles, and death.

A few years later, Tony and I had the privilege to serve together in Mexico City. This massive city of 24 million inhabitants provided us an opportunity to do church planting together, while working in garbage dumps that were home to displaced people of Central and South America. It was our constant routine to walk in the midst of filth, yet providing comfort to a destitute people who were faceless wanderers lost in an overpopulated metropolis.

Having high levels of pollution, Mexico City's air was not kind to our lungs. After working and walking all day, we would come back and collapse in our one bedroom house. Often, I would see Tony sleep for hours. I supposed that the change of elevation, the tiresome public transport into the city, and the unhealthy food we were eating had something to do with his constant headaches and fatigue.

After serving in Mexico City for awhile, we returned to Texas to recuperate before our next assignment. Our bodies must have gone into shock when we began to breathe healthy air and drank cleaner water. We coughed for weeks as our lungs began to filter themselves. It was during this time that it happened. Tony would sleep for long hours again without having true rest. In the middle of the night, he work up with a massive headache and was rushed to the hospital. It was then that the diagnosis was given. Tony had a brain tumor.

The Hand of Providence

"…and to God the Lord belong escapes from death."

—Psalm 68:20

It was1971. I was barely 2 months old. As I traveled in my mother's arms on Highway 89 en route to San Francisco, an oncoming car came out of nowhere, lost control and slammed into our vehicle. Of course, being so young, I remember nothing of the incident; but my mother says it was a "milagro de Dios" that I was not crushed to death. Both cars were a total loss. My mother was knocked unconscious. Miraculously, I ended up slipping below the steering wheel instead of being crushed to death by it. Incredibly, I was remarkably unharmed. This was not to be the only time I was to face death as a young child.

Later on in my childhood, my family took an extended vacation into the interior of Mexico. I experienced major culture shock as we stopped in a tiny pueblito and were faced with the limited facilities of a third world country. The things I previously seen as life's necessities—proper running water to drink and wash with, sanitary restrooms, and local medical help—were nowhere to be found in this God-forsaken little town. I contractd some form of cholera, probably from the unsanitary conditions. I eventually recovered. But even then my encounters with death were by no means over.

My next brush with the Angel of Death came when I was around 11 years old. It was during the Passover holiday, when my family and I were enjoying a customary gathering of relatives at a local park located on the Rio Grande River. It was a sunny afternoon; the water looked inviting and the currents seemed peaceful. I was intrigued to see some older men swimming back and forth across the Rio.Grande Curious, I decided to try it myself. Once in the water, however, I found myself battling currents that were far more powerful than I ever imagined. Overcome by the force of the water, I began sinking rapidly. In desperation, I screamed for help with my last breath, and then sank beneath the waters. Within minutes, someone pulled me out of the deep waters and began performing CPR. God had spared me once again. Then, in my unsaved state, I could not see the Hand of God. But now, as a child of God, I can only be thankful that His goodness kept me from drowning, thus saving me from an eternity of damnation. But the enemy was still not finished trying to take my life!

The fourth time the Lord intervened and kept me from dying was during a spring break trip with my cross country teammates to South Padre Island in 1987. One particular evening a friend and I decided to go for a motorcycle ride to pass the time. We realized too late, however, that we had somehow found ourselves driving on a road that was under construction. The front wheel of the bike struck the high side of the road, throwing the bike into an uncontrollable skid. Before either of us could react, we were flung from the bike and onto the road. The impact of my head on the pavement was so great that it cracked the helmet in half! As amazing as it seems, a minor headache and a few insignificant cuts and bruises were the extent of my injuries. My friend was also spared any serious damage. Fortunately, since we had actually been thrown into the other lane, there were no oncoming cars. Once again, I was spared from any serious consequences. It was only later I discovered that few people survive motorcycle accidents like we experienced, let alone just walk away with no serious injuries. God was surely merciful.

The Hand of Providence was upon me.

Champions Are Made

"He has made everything beautiful in its time. Also, He has put eternity in their hearts."

—Ecclesiastes 3:11

As I grew older and became more reflective about life in general, I found my mind wandering through these incidents. I began to consider why I hadn't died in any of these situations. While anyone could have a "lucky day", and walk away from a potentially dangerous situation unscathed, I had survived several incidents—any one of which could have (actually, should have) taken my life. I could not escape a nagging suspicion that these incidents meant something, but being raised in a non-Christian environment, I had no clue what that "something" might be. The thought that the answer was a Someone instead of a something never crossed my mind, let alone the idea that this "Someone" might have a "future and a hope" especially for me.

The thought of God and religion had always turned me off; yet I had many questions that refused to go away. As much as I would have preferred not to, I found myself thinking about them. What would it take for me to make it to heaven? Where did I come from? What was I doing here on earth? I had not been satisfied by following the empty traditions of Catholicism practiced by my culture, they left me puzzled and empty. What was the point of performing elaborate, spiritual rituals if they only left you spiritually dead? To me, it seemed like having a fast and beautiful car, but no gas to run it.

In his book "Eternity In Their Hearts", author Don Richardson tells us that God has placed a sense of eternity in all people. I was no exception. I grew up in the barrio, and by the time I was in middle school, I had been exposed to just about everything there is to know about drugs and crime. I never imagined that some of the friends I grew up with would end up serving life sentences for murder; but, somehow, I did have a deep desire to try and make sense of the meaningless life of hatred and unlawfulness that surrounded me in the barrio. This quest for meaning led me to a desperate attempt to find a way out of the barrio. Being somewhat athletic, I figured that sports would be a good avenue out of a rough life. In 1983 I joined both the cross country and track teams at my school, two sports that seemed strangely appropriate for me, given my background. Now, instead of running away from the police like I was used to doing, I was running with no one chasing me but the other kids on the track team. I figured if I was going to be running, I may as well run for my school and get some recognition for it.

But I quickly found out that there is a big difference between a short sprint through an alley and over a fence and a cross-country race. My first years running in middle school were years of hard work learning persistence, determination, and most importantly, how to suffer defeat. I did not win one race in those two years. (So much for gaining recognition!) As a result, the greatest thing I learned was the art of humility! I was not born a gifted runner, but I was determined to stick with it and finish.

For pretty much the remainder of my years in high school, the sport of running (plus a brief foray into the cult religion of Mormonism—more on that later) became my religion. Although my coach encouraged me to join football rather than cross country because I was not physically fit (go figure!), in my heart I knew that through determination, a positive attitude, long hours of exercise and a nutritious diet, I could develop into a competent runner.

"Be a champion in practice; that is where champions are made." This motto inspired me throughout my running years. Some people think that success comes easily in running; however, nothing could be further from the truth. In cross-country racing, as in every other sport, champions are not "born"; they are made, through hours of grueling practice.

And there were literally hours of practice. Despite my coach's discouragement, I believed in my heart that I could succeed. Belief became determination, and determination gave way to obsession. Yes, I was obsessed; and nothing could hold me back from reaching my goal. Since my coach didn't believe in me, I had to create an effective program to train myself. The training was often difficult and often times lonesome; but I had adopted the attitude of a self-motivator. This "religion" of self-achievement, expressed for me by mile after mile of running, filled an empty place inside me; and I went after it with all my heart. I continued to press myself, eventually getting to the point where I was running an average distance of forty miles per week. Along with this, I was doing aerobic swimming several days a week as a means of cardiovascular conditioning. This also massaged my muscles and helped relax them after the rigorous workouts I put myself through.

I gave myself no rest. Even during the off-season and vacation times, I continued to practice. During the Christmas holidays I held myself to a special schedule, running both mornings and evenings. I forced myself to wake up at 5:30 a.m., rain or shine, hot or cold, and run six miles. In the evening, my workout included a combination of mile repetitions, fartlek (this type of training consists of a balance between speed distance and jogging distance. For example if you sprint 100 meters then you counter with 100 meters of jogging. If you sprint 200 meters than you counter jogging 200 meters. The workout tends to last thirty to forty-five minutes.), and speed distance running. During the summers from 1985 to 1989, I participated in the U.S.A. Junior Olympics Program. I was determined to improve my personal time, and I as taking every avenue I could find to shave a few seconds where I could. I even supplemented my race conditioning with weight training; but only in the off-season, to avoid any injuries that would keep me out of competition. Perhaps my coach didn't believe in me, but at least I had come to believe in myself. If I didn't win a race, I was determined that it would not be because of a lack of stamina or out-of-shape muscles. Knowing the strength I had developed gave me confidence upon my return to regular school practice sessions.

In addition to physical training, my eating habits played a major role in my success as an athlete. I learned to eat foods rich in carbohydrates, which not only increased my body's energy, but helped my metabolism. I often forced myself to eat large amounts of lasagna and spaghetti. I avoided drinks that contained caffeine and other irritating chemicals that can cause headaches, high blood pressure and a host of other complications when overused. "Why not stick to milk?" I assured myself that, after all, it promises to "do the body good!" I drank lots of bottled water, juice, and milk. Alcohol, cigarettes and illicit drugs were completely out of the question; I needed my lungs (as well as the rest of my body) in tip-top shape if I was going to be able to perform well. This "discovery" of the power of good eating habits was to influence me greatly later in life as I went through the rigors of chemotherapy.

Mental preparation was an equally important ingredient in my training. I constantly told myself that the extra practice would give me an advantage over my competitors. I found a sense of freedom that I couldn't find anywhere else when I was running. There's nothing quite like the rush of adrenaline pumping through your body. I loved it, goose bumps and all,. There was a simplicity in running. On the track, I didn't have to rely on anyone but me. I only had to be strong, work hard, and strive for excellence. I could block out the world around me and focus. Running, and the disciplines involved in it, gave me a structure in which I could analyze the things going on in my life, make sense of my problems and overcome (so I thought) any obstacle.

I can still remember the day I found myself on the starting line of the Texas State High School/University Interscholastic League's cross country meet. I remember taking pride in the work that had brought me there. I reflected on the hard physical work I had gone through to get there. The hours of practice. The countless miles. Foolishly, I felt as though I could do anything. Looking back today on all that God allowed me to do, I believe with all my heart that He used those very disciplines I learned on the practice track to prepare me, physically as well as mentally, for the fiery trial that only He knew awaited me. He truly does know the plans He has for us. He never allows a situation to enter our lives without giving us exactly what we need to pass through it in complete victory.

Since we're talking about foolish pride, I will admit to being very proud as I finished High School about proving my former coach wrong in the end. By the time I graduated from high school, I had earned the chance to compete in one National Junior Olympics cross country meet and two Texas State High School cross country meets, where I made the final round both years. Not only that, but I was awarded not one but four full scholarships from various universities around the country. Sometimes success does not come overnight, but when it came, it sure was sweet! I obviously had a ways to go in developing humility, but I had not let him hold me down.

On The Road To Damascus

"And when we all had fallen on the ground, I heard a voice speaking to me, saying in the Hebrew language, 'Saul, Saul, why are you persecuting Me?' So I said, 'Who are you, Lord?' I am Jesus, whom you are persecuting. But rise and stand on your feet, for I have appeared to you for this purpose, to make you a minister and a witness of the things which you have seen and of the things I will reveal to you.'"

—Acts 26:12

In the fall of 1988, I had just finished competing at the Texas U.I.L. 5-A High School Cross Country State Meet in Austin, Texas. Little did I know that my life was about to be changed forever. Up to this point, my high school years had been so full of running, competing, studying, and then resting up from all of the above that I hardly ever took time for any of the usual "going out" things that many of my high school friends enjoyed. Weekend leisure time was out of the question for me; Saturdays were competition days, and Sundays were spent catching up on homework, studying for tests or simply resting. At any rate, I always had an excuse—and a good one!—to avoid activities that held no appeal for me.

One such activity was the Mission High School student Bible study. However, I hadn't counted on the persistence of one Alex Sanders, a fellow student and sold-out Christian. I was struck by Alex' perseverance, friendliness, and passion, though I really had no idea what made him so very excited about this Bible study. His numerous invitations were met by my half-hearted promises to attend "soon, when the cross country season is over" which I forgot as soon as I hung up the phone. But though I was willing to forget, Alex was not. I finally came to the conclusion that the "preacher boy" wouldn't let me rest until he saw me walk through the doors to the Bible study Thursday mornings.

Though the odds were against our developing a friendship, somehow it happened. I perceived Alex as a middle-class yuppie sort of person, with a culture and world-view far removed from my tough barrio upbringing. I was suspicious of his motives for befriending me. Now I know it was his commitment to pray for me

7

that broke down the barriers between us. But break them down he did, allowing Alex and I to establish enough of a friendship that I was willing to spend some time with him. I guess that was why it didn't seem strange when Alex invited me to sleep over at his house…on a Wednesday night. Talk about strategic evangelism! Before I knew it, the "trap" had sprung. By the time I realized what was happening, there was no way I could back out. The next morning his father drove us to school—and the Thursday morning Bible study!

Throughout the meeting, there was singing, clapping, shouting and a message given from the Bible; all with no interference whatsoever from the school administration. At first I thought, "Who are these people and what exactly are they promoting?" I questioned whether they were for real, or if this was just a well-constructed front they were putting on for my benefit. Yet even as questions and doubts were running through my mind, I could not escape the sense that there was something different, something deeper going on in the lives of these students. I noted that there were young people from different backgrounds, different economic levels, various parts of town and all walks of life, and they were here together. They actually seemed to be accepting one another. They were full of peace, and joy and something else I couldn't quite put my finger on. Now I know it was Jesus, and the love that comes from knowing Him, plain and simple. I didn't recognize that love, because I had never known a love like that before. But even though I had no words to describe what I saw they all had, by the end of the meeting I knew I wanted it—whatever "it" was. I found out that the "it" was actually a "Him". When the call was made for those who desired to commit their lives to Christ Jesus to step forward, I went and yielded my life, my dreams, my reputation and my soul to Him.

◆   ◆   ◆

In the following weeks, my commitment to Jesus grew. God and His Holy Spirit were not done introducing themselves to me. I sensed there was more, much more, to my new walk with Christ, but I wasn't sure what that "more" was. As the weeks grew into months, it became clear that the Great Physician would have to perform a lot of "spiritual surgery" in my own spirit. It would take the ministry of the Holy Spirit to bestow His comfort and conviction in the areas of my life that needed healing and cleansing.

In time, this knowledge led me to seek the infilling of the Holy Spirit. I prayed to receive the Holy Spirit, just as I had read about in the Book of Acts. Amazingly, I received a double portion of His grace and mercy, and as I did, I heard the words "Whoever is ashamed of Me and My words in front of men, of him the Son of man will be ashamed when He comes in His glory" (Luke 8:38). I knew then and there that God was calling me into the ministry as a missionary. Though I was only newly graduated from high school, I wasted no time in making the necessary preparations to enter the ministry. But just as quickly as I determined to follow and obey, obstacles arose to hinder my plans.

The first issue to arise was academic. I had made a commitment to attend a certain college on a full athletic scholarship, and was scheduled to begin college that coming fall. I was convinced that it was the Lord's will for me to give up the scholarship. I believed that He wanted me to start my ministerial training right away, and to do so on a full time basis. Much to my surprise, not only my family but also many in my own congregation criticized my desire to do this. In fact, there were even some in my church who actually wagged their fingers in my face and told me I was foolish to give up a free education. They told me that I had been given a once-in-a-lifetime chance at the American Dream, and accused me of foolishly throwing it all away.

I wasn't sure if they were right or not. But I was sure that Jesus had said He would use the foolish things of the world to confound the wise. I was convinced in my heart of this one thing: God had called me to serve Him in preaching the Gospel. If serving Him meant that he wanted me to give up a free education, I knew that the Lord had a valid reason.

The second obstacle came in the form of my mother. She refused to give her blessing to my plan to attend a Youth With A Mission discipleship program in Tyler, Texas instead of starting college. I was convinced that the YWAM program was part of God's plan for me, yet I felt it would be wrong to go against the directly command of one of the primary authorities God had placed in my life: my mother. It was here that I was to learn a valuable lesson about the power of submission and prayer!

Even though things looked hopeless as far as Mom ever changing her mind, I continued to pray about the situation. I felt that I was supposed to quietly continue to prepare for the YWAM school. I applied for and was accepted into their Discipleship Training Program. During the summer I worked two full-time jobs, one at McDonalds and the other at a local Boy's and Girl's Club. On my days off, I worked odd jobs as well. By the end of the summer, I had raised enough money to pay my full tuition for the YWAM program. I had the desire, the call and the money; but I still didn't have my mother's permission to go.

Throughout this entire time, I pleaded with the Lord to move in my mother's heart. I knew I could not go without her permission and her blessing. The Bible says in Proverbs 21:1 that the king's heart is in God's hand. Evidently Mom's hearts are in His hand, too. After three long months, He answered my prayer and my Mom gave her blessing. Thank you, Jesus! God made a way!

Upon my arrival at the Youth With A Mission headquarters in Lindale, Texas, my emotions were running high. I never imagined I would find a missionary school in the middle of nowhere, much less on a ranch. Yet even in the midst of the barren land I could sense God's presence and peace in that place. Over the next six months, I would find myself on the Potter's wheel, my character and relationship with Jesus being molded and shaped by God and His various "tools". More than external skills to be learned, there was a lot of inner healing to be done, as well. There was a great deal of unforgiveness I had to deal with as I continued my growth in the Lord. I found the teachings on the Father's Heart of God were some of the most crucial, actually changing my whole concept of God as my Heavenly Father. The Bible teaches in Psalm 27:10 "When my father and mother forsake me, then the Lord will take care of me." Having been raised without a father figure, the concept of God as a father was incomprehensible. However, I knew that in order to mature in God's ways, my past could not have a negative effect upon my present and future walk with my Heavenly Father. In order to trust, love and serve God, my devotion to him would have to be one of clean hands and a pure heart. In essence, my devotional time with him was a direct response of my concept of God. The yearning of the Holy Spirit was strong and at work in my life that I knew I could come and rest under the shadow of his wings.

As I continued to trust God by having an appreciation for his character, I realized that no good thing would earn me his favor, but assurance and confidence to trust him more. I chose to lean solely on Isaiah 55:8 His thoughts are not my thoughts neither his ways my ways.

I could only fathom of coming to the cross and dying to self that I may be purified by his blood. God was more interested in the condition of my heart than in any rituals or Theology. During those precious months at YWAM, I learned what it meant to be drawn by the Holy Spirit to times of prayer, fasting, and reading His word. I began to see how the disciplines I had developed during my years of running might now be of benefit in the kingdom of God. I experienced times of laughter, weeping, confusion, pain, isolation—and revelation. During my time in Discipleship Training School I learned several valuable lessons that no one can ever take away, truths that guide my walk with the Lord to this day. In February of 1990, I completed the program. A transformed person, I returned to

Mission, Texas with plans to enter the ministry internship program "Last Days Harvesters" at my local church.

That March I entered the program as a missionary intern. I knew that there would be a lot to learn about people, service, and character. As an intern staff missionary, I had to learn servanthood. Some of the duties that helped in this education were running errands, painting walls, and cleaning toilets! In my heart, I was thrilled to do anything if it was for Jesus.

During the summer months I was in charge of food preparation for the youth groups that stayed at our church during short term missions outreaches to Mexico. The work was enormous, but it was worth it all to see the lost in Mexico come to Jesus, and to see the lives of the youth being challenged and their faith deepened as they served in this way.

That winter I was allowed to serve as the co-leader of a group of young people on a missionary outreach to Barcelona, Spain, where we assisted some local church planters in evangelizing their territory. The next summer I was in Mexico City, Mexico, where I would later return to serve with an Career Missionary missionary previously stationed there. While on this assignment, I was able to pastor some of the young people of that city as well as assisting the missionary in his church-planting endeavors. Upon returning from Mexico, the Lord allowed me to go Singapore and Malaysia to work with other young people. My heart was being stirred for the many peoples of the world who had not yet heard the good news of Jesus Christ; I desired to bring them into the kingdom of God, whatever the cost, and my goal was to learn as much as I could from the intern program in order to fulfill that desire.

One of the steps I felt the Lord was leading me to take was to continue my Biblical studies via the correspondence program provided by my church and to pursue ministerial credentials. At first, it felt awkward to be back in Bible school after so much hands-on work in the field. I completed several courses and was able to receive my Christian worker's license. Another two years of study allowed me to meet the requirements for a full licensed to minister. The study and preparation continued, and my goal of full ordination was realized on April 18, 1996.

Surprised By Cancer

"These things I have spoken unto you, that in Me you may have peace. In the world you will have tribulation; but be of good cheer, for I have overcome the world."

—John 16:33

I can certainly relate to these words spoken by Jesus Christ in the Gospel of John. The word "tribulation" is defined as anguish, burden and trouble. My tribulation came in the form of a completely unexpected battle with cancer.

In January of 1992, I was rushed to the McAllen Medical Center with an incredible pain in my head. I was admitted immediately, and within 3 hours received the diagnosis that would change my life. the doctor's told me that I had an astrocytoma—a brain tumor. In the shock of the moment, I had no idea of the implications of this diagnosis. Amazingly, even in the midst of that horrible situation, I experienced an immediate, deep peace within. I had the Holy Spirit's assurance that everything was in God's hands. As the diagnosis was pronounced "it's a brain tumor", immediately the Holy Spirit told me "Tony everything is going to be fine, don't fret." Having realized that the word "fear" conveys false evidence that appear real, I simply allowed the Holy Spirit to comfort me with the peace of God that surpasses all understanding.

In a few short moments I became more familiar with the details of astrocytoma tumors than I ever thought I would become. I learned that they are usually found either around the brain or spinal column, and can be either benign or malignant. In my case, my tumor had embedded itself in my brain. It was malignant, which meant that it was expected to spread; becoming progressively worse and life-threatening. An emergency operation had to be performed. It lasted over eight hours.

After a nine hour surgery, I recall hearing the voices of the medical team on the way to the MRI facility. By the time I was placed on the bed of the conductor, I was feeling the effects of the anesthesia wearing off. Feeling a sense of desperation and nervousness, I wondered what was next for me. I felt claustrophobic inside the MRI tunnel. If I dared move one inch, the whole test would have to be done all over from the start. After that exam, I was taken to the intensive care unit. It was here that I would spend the next twenty-one days battling for my life.

From the very beginning of my time in the intensive care unit, I experienced severe complications. After brain surgery, patients face the risk of going into convulsions as a result of the brain going into shock. In my case, that was exactly what happened. I began to experience unpredictable and severe seizures. I was forced to spend long hours with a dry mouth, because my doctors were concerned about fluid going up to the brain and producing even more severe complications. So I was only allowed crushed ice in small portions. At other times, I found it incredibly hard to breathe, as though my brain had somehow forgotten how. Sometimes the combination of the seizures and the inability to breathe made me feel as if I was going to die.

Unknown to me, my condition was steadily worsening. My family, fiancée, and pastor were told that I would probably not survive. The doctor's suggested that it would probably be wise to begin considering funeral arrangements. The best hope they offered to my loved ones was that, if I survived, I would most likely end up in a vegetative state for the rest of my life.

Naturally, I knew none of this. For me, the worst part was that I often felt totally alone. As I lay there, I couldn't help thinking of the cancer battles I would still have to face if I survived the surgery. I compared them with all the plans I had made for ministry. Try as I might, I could find no answers. I could only lay my life at the feet of Jesus. Nothing but my hope in Him was sure; He was the only thing I had to hold on to.

And, thankfully, Jesus was still in control of the whole situation.

Spiritual Warfare

"For though we walk in the flesh, we do not war according to the flesh. For the weapons of our warfare are not carnal but mighty in God for pulling down strongholds."

—2 Corinthians 10:3-4

"Many are the afflictions of the righteous, but the Lord delivers him out of them all."

—Psalm 34:19

One evening, while my fiancée was allowed a visit, something incredible happened. I realize that the conversation I am about to relate to you will sound foolish to those who do not accept the present day ministry of the Holy Spirit, and therefore do not believe in healings, deliverances, or miracles. Perhaps my experience will allow you to reconsider your position.

My fiancée was sitting beside my bed, silently praying for me. The Holy Spirit miraculously woke me up from a medication-induced sleep. I awoke asking Carol to call the pastors at church. She was to tell them that, somehow, the church members were praying wrong.

In awe, Carol replied, "Are you sure you know what you are talking about?"

"Yes," I replied. "You need to tell the church and the ministry staff to pray against and bind a deaf and dumb spirit."

As I said the last word, I fell instantly back asleep. Carol could hardly believe what she had just heard. In her mind, she thought it was probably the result of all the books that I had read on healing by authors such as Kathryn Kuhlman, T.L. Osborn, A. B. Simpson, John G. Lake and John Wimber. Still, there was something about the conversation she simply could not dismiss. She went home and immediately contacted the pastor and related the incident.

I often wonder how many Christians actually follow up on their commitment to pray after receiving a prayer request from someone. In this case, the pastor and staff could have ignored Carol's strange request. Instead, a prayer vigil was called for that night. The pastoral staff, armed with specific instructions from on high, committed to pray through the night for my deliverance from a deaf and dumb spirit, binding it in the Name of Jesus. It was their spiritual warfare, fought throughout that long night, that set me free from the uncontrollable seizures I was having and the possibility of brain damage.

No sooner had we won one battle than another crested the horizon. Many years before coming to Christ, I had made a brief excursion into the cult religion of Mormonism. Now, it came back to haunt me. I did not realize it at the time, but this decision had allowed the enemy of my soul to gain a foothold in my life. Since some Christians are ignorant of the reality of spiritual warfare, I will try to convey what went on during that prayer vigil. I realize that this may sound somewhat bizarre, but it is true none the less.

As the church staff prayed that night, their prayers did reach heaven. They were intent on winning this battle, but they had no idea that by stirring the devil's nest, they were first going to see the spiritual warfare intensified. The reports the staff shared later sounded like scenes that could have been deleted from the movie "The Shining" as too strange to be beleieved. But this was not some Hollywood special effects session, it was in fact a matter of life and death. While the pastors were praying that night, doors through out the church flew open and slammed shut by themselves. In some church offices, books and other objects flew across the room.

In the spirit realm, one of the staff members actually saw a demon hovering over my bed trying to kill me. It was the demon they had been told to bind and cast out, the spirit deaf and dumb spirit. The staff focused their prayers against the evil spirit. Afterwards, another member of the staff was given a vision, and saw the face of one of the leaders in the Mormon movement. Thought these prayer warriors had no idea of my previous involvement with the Mormons, they were shown by the Lord that they needed to take authority over that area, too.

The Holy Spirit moved profoundly through this battle of prayer. Finally, His anointing broke the back of Satan and his cohort. The Holy Spirit's strategy to pray and bind a deaf and dumb spirit was effective. My condition began to turn around that very morning. On the morning following the all-night battle of prayer, I began my recovery. True, it was a recovery that would take lots of patience, work and physical therapy, but it was one that never should have happened in the first place if one holds to the original opinion of the doctors.

Jesus had fulfilled His promise from the first day, when He told me that there was nothing to fear because He was in control. The peace of God that surpasses all understanding had kept my heart in peace, knowing that it was the Lord's battle, not mine. It was His battle, His blood, His power, and His authority that set me free! Free indeed! Upon being released from the hospital I knew that treatments and therapy were sure to follow in the coming months. Carol and I were engaged around the same time that I was diagnosed with cancer, and had to postpone our wedding plans for an estimated year. As the year went by, I continued my recovery while Carol focused on our future plans. Furthermore, I remained isolated from full time ministry as a result of having to endure radiation treatments not to mention physical therapy being that I was paralyzed on my left side. In essence I kept my focus on God's word and prayer seeking his guidance. After all the dust had settled, Carol and I officially had set a date for our wedding. On December 5, 1992, we were married in our home church with family and friends.

Jehovah Jireh

Three months after my surgery, I began a six week treatment of radiation therapy designed to kill any remaining cancer cells in my brain. I found it was embarrassing to go out in public. People could not help staring at my bald head and scarred scalp. "Well," I told myself, "it's just part of the price I have to pay to make sure the cancer doesn't come back." I wish I had been right.

Just one short year later, in September of 1993, I was diagnosed with a recurrence of the tumor. This was an enormous blow and left me with an unbearable sense of desperation. Not only was my health a concern, but by now the devastating reality of the financial burden my sickness was creating was inescapable. My only thought was that this was another opportunity to trust God fully. As Paul described in second Corinthians 1:9 "I had the sentence of death, that I should not trust in myself, but in God who raises the dead." A month before my initial diagnosis of cancer, my health insurance had expired. Not knowing what was to come, I was in no hurry to contact my agent to renew it. But now, my medical bills were piling up, and the pile was growing daily.

Just my first surgery, hospital stay, and radiation therapy expenses had reached a grand total of $65,000. The surgery and therapy had weakened me to the point where I was confined to 24-hour bed-rest, completely unable to work. I felt useless and hopeless. I tried every avenue I could find to get financial assistance, but somehow always fell through the cracks of the bureaucracy. I was unable to get any assistance, and I felt betrayed by the government I'd faithfully served by paying taxes and working for the community.

My financial burden grew by another $30,000 as I underwent a second surgery at M. D. Anderson Cancer Center in Houston, Texas. It was another cancer—expected to spread and getting progressively worse. After the surgery, I was told that I needed to undergo chemotherapy treatments for the next two years. Two Years!! It sounded like an eternity. I had no health insurance, no income, and a financial burden that had grown to somewhere around $85,000. In the natural, there was no hope.

Yet in my heart, I knew I had to hold on to what the Holy Spirit had spoken to me. In spite of what I could see, I had to trust that everything was in God's hands. I had to!!! It was all I had to hold on to, and, by His grace, I was not about to deviate from His promise. I had to believe that, somehow, God would prove faithful to His name. He had said that He was "Jehovah Jireh," my Provider. It was His problem, not mine.

I clearly remember the day that, finally strong enough to get out of bed, I went back to McAllen Medical Center to make an arrangement about the payment of my medical fees from my first hospital stay, surgery and radiation. As I approached the business office, I knew it would be an astronomical amount of money. I felt as though I would end up making monthly payments to them for the rest of my life. The lady behind the counter at the Business Office asked me to take a seat while she pulled up my records and financial information on her computer screen. When she finally reviewed all the information, she told me that the hospital administration had decided to write off the entire amount of $65,000. In my heart, I knew that God had touched the hearts of these people.

At the M.D. Anderson Hospital in Houston, my balance was close to $30,000. Since the neurologist on my case there hoped that I would be a candidate for a clinical trial—a non-surgical laser procedure for brain tumors—he went ahead and made all the necessary arrangements for me to be treated at M. D. Anderson. The ironic thing was that their least concern was the money to pay for this expensive surgery. After the three hour procedure and a night in the hospital, I was on my way to a full recovery with no complications. In the weeks that followed, I called the Center to inquire about my bill, and once again, was told on the phone that I had a zero balance. My entire billI on the computer had been deleted. They had no record of me owing the hospital a penny! Just to be sure, I asked the lady to please send me something on paper, to keep as proof. I still have the receipt for that zero balance. Once again, God had proven faithful.

However there was still the expense of my chemotherapy treatments and the numerous flights I would have to take from the home to Houston to receive them. Of course the money didn't arrive through the sky or by mail. But once again, the Lord moved in authority over my bills. But by the time I needed to start the chemotherapy, an anonymous person had donated airline tickets for me to use for the entire length of my treatments in Houston.

God's favor and faithfulness were so evident—I kept remembering the promise He had given me since day one and proceeded to do what had to be done. Many aspects of my life changed dramatically. While undergoing the chemo, I simply didn't have the strength to run my customary six miles a day. The changes in my life and diet were often time-consuming and inconvenient. My physician advised me to avoid caffeine, dairy products, acids and all varieties of red meat.

Instead I was to eat all natural foods that were rich in protein and included fresh fruits, vegetables and grains. This put a lot of pressure on my wife, Carol, as she had to cook—no fast food!—three or four meals daily in addition to putting in a ten hour day at work. There was hardly any time to just enjoy being together. I felt guilty for not being able to do my share of the housekeeping.

◆   ◆   ◆

Cancer has changed the way I looked at the world, both literally and figuratively. I lost my left peripheral vision as a result of the first surgery. I still use extreme caution in driving because of this. After the second surgery I was told that I would need to undergo chemotherapy treatments. During the first stages of my treatments, the oncologist that I was seeing at the time took it upon himself to change the protocol prescribed by Dr.'s at M.D. Anderson, resulting in a chemo overdose, leaving me in a state of shock for about 48hrs. I've also had to quit participating in weekend football and basketball games with my friends. At times this has made me feel like I don't really "belong" with my friends anymore, like the cancer has made me different. But at the same time, being able to drive, hold a job, and attend a university have become precious treasures to me, things that many have taken for granted. For me, they are miracles in a life that has been filled with miracles.

The tribulations I've faced as a result of the cancer have been many and varied, hitting me not only in the physical realm, but in my emotions, relationships, finances and spirituality. Only because of my close relationship to my Lord and Savior Jesus Christ have I been able to overcome these critical phases.

The School Of Suffering

"For to you it has been granted on behalf of Christ, not only to believe in Him, but also to suffer for His sake...."

—Philippians 1:29

I don't profess to know everything there is to know about the subject of suffering. I do know, however, what it's like to battle brain cancer for seven years, and I have experienced first-hand physical, spiritual, and emotional pain, as well as the pain of those who surrounded me with their love and support during that time. God has graciously allowed me to pass through the school of suffering.

Whatever trial you may find yourself in, God is able, if you allow Him, to use that time to refine your faith and draw you closer to Himself. As a believer in Christ I chose to put on the whole armor of God, as Paul instructed in the scriptures, and got a solid grip on the truth of God's word. God is a God that swore by His own name, that His word would not return to Him void.

One of the first battles I had to face was against the lies of rejection. In the days before Jesus came to earth, the Jewish people had their own philosophy of the purpose of suffering. They believed that, when people experienced trials and tribulations, it was because of sin that was in their lives. Suffering was the judgment of God that had come upon them. A corollary to that was that, if one was being blessed and prospering, then the favor of God was upon him. We are still so tempted to listen to the lies of the devil. He whispers, quite convincingly, that God doesn't love us anymore, that His judgment is upon us for our sinful life. During the early hours of my diagnosis as I laid in my hospital bed, several visitors had the audacity to ask me if I was living in sin. Although I was appalled by these remarks, I could only think of Job and how he faced a similar situation as this. My focus was not on being defensive, but rather on standing on the promises of God.

This, of course, is completely contrary to the doctrine of our salvation and the Word of God. Jesus came and took the judgment we deserve, and give us the blessing we don't deserve. As if that wasn't enough, we have God's assurance in His word that He truly is on our side:

"What then shall we say to these things? If God is for us, who can be against us?" Romans 8:31. "When I cry out to You, then my enemies will turn back; this I know, because God is for me." Psalm 56:9.

Another lesson I had to learn concerns an old philosophical argument. "How can a good God could allow evil things to happen to His people?" We have believers among us who once positively glowed with the joy of the Lord, but are now embittered, perhaps back-slidden, blinded and unable to grow because they are holding a grudge against God. Sometimes this bitterness against God is so severe they abandon their faith entirely. During the outreach to Barcelona, Spain, when I was a missionary intern, I encountered a man who claimed to be an atheist. After spending some time witnessing to him, he mentioned that he used to be a born-again Christian. However, when the times of testing and difficulty came his way, he blamed God for them. From that time on, he wanted nothing more to do with Christianity.

In spite of going through times of suffering, believers should remember that God is not the author of evil:" For You are not a God who takes pleasure in wickedness." (Psalm 5:4). Because of the fall of man, evil is permitted, but it is not something in which God takes pleasure. We must not forget that He causes "all things to work together for good to those who love God, to those who are called according to His purpose." (Romans 8:28).

One of the most important things God will teach us in the school of suffering, if we allow it, is the state of our own hearts. In fact, God is much more concerned about that than He is about delivering us from our trial. The trial is taking place in this physical realm, which will eventually pass away. But our heart is with us through eternity. In Psalms 4:4 we are instructed to "meditate within your heart on your bed, and be still." In the midst of trials and suffering, the Christian has an excellent opportunity to search and judge their own hearts. You may find yourself grappling with some heavy questions. Will I only love Him when things are going great? Will I only love Him when I feel His presence? Will I only love Him when I get my own way? If so, then is this really love?

We all know those who prayed diligently for their miracle of healing, got it, thanked Jesus, and never entered a church again. They forfeit the potential that was in them to be a vessel of God and minister to others in their time of trouble. In John 6, Jesus fed the multitudes and did many miracles., Yet many walked away after their needs were met. Jesus asked the remaining disciples if they wanted to leave as well. May all of our answers be as Simon Peter's: "Lord, to whom shall we go? You alone have the words of eternal life." (John 6:68).

Running the Race

"Know ye not that they which run in a race run all, but one receiveth the prize? So run, that ye may obtain."

—I Corinthians 9:24

In Philippians 2:15, Paul also reminds believers to "hold fast to the word of life…that we might not run in vain." As I reflect on my battle with cancer, the trophies, medals and plaques that I ran countless miles to win seem to fade into the background. None of these accomplishments really matter in the end. Only the healing power of God remains. During my trips to M. D. Anderson Cancer Center, I felt a deep compassion for the victims around me. Many of the patients I came into contact with had no hope. If we're to run the race Paul has called us to run—if we're to be champions for Christ—we must resolve these issues regardless of the battles we are engaged in.

The devil may lie to you in the midst of your situation, telling you, "God must not love you very much if He's letting this happen to you."

Please allow me to encourage you to find truth in what the Bible proclaims.

1st Corinthians 9:24 "Do you not know that those who run in a race will run, but only one receives the prize? Run in such a way that you may obtain it. And everyone who competes for the prize is temperate in all things. Now they do it to obtain a perishable crown, but we for an imperishable crown.

As a former distance runner in Cross Country and Track, these thought-provoking words by the Apostle Paul, are crucial in order to finish the race the Lord Jesus Christ has called us to run. Although the life of a runner is lonesome, hard work, three hundred and sixty five days a year, allow me to take you into the mind, soul, and body of a runner who desires to be a Champion. I do not give you a vain philosophy, but basic principles that drove me from a reject in my early years of running to my God-given potential and destiny.

"I DON'T BELIVE IN DEFEAT!"

- Do you allow the devil to deceive you, rather than Jesus to lead you in victory.
- Greater is he that is in you that he that is in the world. 1 John 4:4
- Realize the easy days of no pressure are over.
- You can't win today on what you did in the last race. (NOTE FOR THE EDITOR: last race, or yesterday).
- You can do all things through Christ who strengthens you. Phil 4:13

"NO PRICE IS TO HIGH TO PAY IN JESUS

- Work on the attitude that says "I can" or "I will" no matter what the odds.
- A reckless abandonment to finish the race.
- Run and work in full capacity daily.
- Don't take pride in merely going to church; this is no achievement.
- We can no longer honor participation; anyone can participate.
- Develop a spirit like Joshua, Caleb, Gideon, and Jesus.

"TO BE A WINNER, WORK HARDER LONGER THAN YOUR ENEMY"

- Is food more important than the Word of God?
- Is fasting a common attribute in your walk to bring down Principalities and Powers.
- Do you pray without ceasing?
- Do you offer token prayers?
- Does Hell recognize your name?

"A CROWN OF LIFE AWAITS THOSE THAT PERSEVERE TO THE END"

- God is more interested in your heart than your talents.

- God is more interested in those who serve than those than can lead.

- God can do more with the one percent totally dedicated than the uncommitted ninety-nine percent.

- God will never allow anything to meet your needs, but he himself.

- God resists the proud, but gives grace to the humble. James 4:6

"WISHFUL THINKING:"

- Won't make you an over comer, but the Blood of Jesus.

- Won't make you a Christian, but knowing Jesus Christ as the savior of your life.

- Must be buried, that we may dwell in those things that are pure, lovely, honest, and of good value.

- Contradicts the Word of God; without faith it is impossible to please God.

- Won't make you a Champion.

"GANAS: THE DESIRE OF A CHAMPION"

- The inner self of man no longer satisfied with the status quo.

- The urgency to change or challenge it's present, past, or future conditions.

- The notion to accomplish the unthinkable despite obstacles.

- Follows those that lead with integrity; not those with titles.

- Recognizes the wisdom and gift from God; Does not boast or lean on the arm of the flesh.

- Makes a runner be on time to practice and proactive rather than reactive.

- Says "yes" when others say it can't be done.

"VITAMINS FOR RUNNERS:

- The key to running lies in more running, and the key to life is hungering for more Jesus.

- The basis for success is hard, diligent work; therefore there is no escape.

- Nothing is ever done half heartedly.
- Nothing really worthwhile has ever been accomplished without enthusiasim.
- With God all things are possible to them that believe.
- The word "QUIT" is never an option.
- Excuses will get you nowhere.

"PAIN"

- You can never achieve greatness without pain.
- Jesus drank his cup of pain.
- Through much tribulation, we will inherit the Kingdom of God.
- It is not enough to believe, but to suffer for His sake.
- The days of easy "believism" are over.

"OVERCOMING"

- Jesus said "Be of good cheer, I have overcome the world". John 16:33
- Champions are not born of people who always have things their way.
- Is a trait that belongs to a Champion.
- An obstacle will either overcome, or be overcome.
- Winners are not those who go through a season and never face a real challenge.
- Jesus Christ knows of our disappointments.
- Jesus faced the ordeal of betrayal, denial, and crucifixion, and overcame it.

Don't quit running "The Race".

Epilogue

"We talk of the second coming, but half the world has never heard of the first." As I read and ponder this thought provoking quote by Oswald J. Smith, I am more than convinced that the Lord Jesus has spared me for His purposes. Although I might have gone through some minor inconveniences, I know the hand of "Providence" is in control. As I bring closure to this time of trial and testing, allow me to bring you up to date with my situation here at the end of the Year of Our Lord 2004.

As I always strive to be pro-active in my endeavors, rather than whining through my ordeals, I took the initiative to pursue a double major in Special Education and Nursing. I am now one semesters away from a scheduled graduation in the fall of 2004. In addition, I am currently in the process of birthing a medical ministry with emphasis on working in Mexico and the "10/40 Window." In essence, since I volunteer as a Youth and Missions Pastor, the Lord has released me to open a Missions School by the name of HATIKVAH School of Missions, International. I have always believed that God's callings are not to be forsaken; therefore, I am indebted to the call of the "Great Commission."

In closing, I pray my testimony would not only bring hope in a Savior that has conquered death, hell, and the grave, but also show that he is faithful and true to his covenant.

Currently, I have been declared in remission from Brain Cancer. I can only speak from what I have experienced, that my God is faithful and able to do exceedingly and abundantly all that he has promised.

Carol: A Wife Coping with Cancer

"How does one cope when their loved one is diagnosed with cancer?"

I say, "Pray, pray, pray and when you're done praying pray some more…"

Webster's Dictionary of the English Language defines "coping" as "a struggle to overcome difficulty". This is exactly what the family of a cancer patient does as they struggle to make sense out of the chaotic circumstances into which they are thrust. When the diagnosis is declared, different family members go through different processes to come to grips with the situation. At the beginning stage, the spouse (and even the patient) are likely experience a sense of trauma. It is not uncommon to ask the question, "Why is this happening?" I have found no suitable answers.

Anxiety and impatience builds when not finding the answers to your questions. Please note that the journey to make sense and assimilate the impact of the illness is a very complex one.

As the spouse of a man who unexpectedly got diagnosed with a malignant tumor, I am compelled to share some strategies that worked for me. My hope and prayers is that my personal experiences will help cancer patients and their loved ones cope with the burdens that a cancer illness produces. As you are aware, cancer does not come with a "how to" manual that will help families cope with the emotional, physical and financial stresses that the illness produces.

"How can I cope with today?" (Let alone tomorrow.) This my friend I learned through heartaches and pains! I had to learn some strategies to survive the horror that the illness was bringing upon my family. That these strategies will help ou I can only hope and pray.

Once the prognosis is handed down, the family has to make decisions on treatments." Always, and I emphasize ALWAYS, get at least three doctor's opinions.

Why? Because three heads are better than two. And with the life of a loved one hanging in the balance, I have found the insight from the third voice to be helpful and reassuring.

Beware! Making treatment decisions can turn into an emotional roller coaster. Be prepared to have some family members disagree with your selection of treatment options! Unfortunately, this may lead to long-term family feuds if you are not careful. Through much prayer, someone in the family has to take authority in assisting the victim make wise decisions. While the patient's spouse should consult the in-laws and other key people, these people need to understand that they are being asked to give an opinion, not render a decision. The cancer victim (and his/her spouse, when there is one) must clearly reserve the right to make the ultimate decision. Everyone will benefit from remembering that time is limited when making decisions related to cancer treatment. It is unwise to waste it on bickering,. Use it to make the best and most informed choice of treatments you can.

Also, research as much as possible on the illness, realizing that you will never have "enough" information. This includes causes, treatment options, recovery procedures and nutrition. At the beginning, you may not even want to see the word cancer or tumor, but you need to overcome this fear! The bible says, "My people perish for a lack of knowledge." So arm yourself with as much information as you can to defeat your enemy! Knowing your enemy will give you insight to ask doctors the appropriate questions. As you go about doing your research and caring for your loved one, be sure to take care of your own emotional and physical needs.

Your emotions are likely to be "hanging on a string". The most insignificant comment from a well-intended friend or family member may send you into a rage. In order to avoid mood swings, you need to get plenty of sleep and eat healthy meals. Sleep deprivation will rob your brain of normal cognitive functions and will cause physical fatigue.

"How can I ensure that we'll eat well balanced meals with the schedule we're going to be facing?"

You may think, it's impossible to prepare healthy meals when you're spending so much time at hospitals and doctors offices. But simply pack a light, non-perishable lunch and take it wherever you go. Prepare ahead of time by shopping for whole wheat breads, bagels, apples, nuts, bottled juices and water that will keep you hydrated and give you plenty of energy. Yes, you do need to take care of yourself before you can take care of anyone else!

Also, I recommend that you adopt a nightly ritual that will help ease anxiety. For example, prepare to go to bed by reading an inspirational book and ending with a short prayer. This will help you turn over your daily burdens to your Heavenly Father. He will give you a sense of freedom and peace that will prepare your body to wind down and have a good night's sleep.

I also suggest that you get your finances in order. I got a spiral notebook and label budget. List all sources of income and tally your monthly total income. Then, list all of your current monthly expenses such as tithe, mortgage, car payments, insurance, utilities, groceries, gas, medical bills, cable television, newspaper subscriptions, etc. Subtract the total monthly expenditures from your total monthly income.

If you are in the red do not panic! It is likely that you can still make ends meet. First, take your needs to the Lord in prayer. Ask Him for wisdom to get you ready to develop a plan to meet your obligations. Begin by setting aside money to pay for non-negotiables such as tithe, mortgage, car and utilities.

The next step is to figure out how much you can pay on the incurred medical bills. Can you pay a few hundred dollars a month for medical expenses? Once you have this information, refer to your list of medical creditors and contact them. Ask to speak with the collections department manager and explain your financial situation and offer an amount that you can pay monthly. Most medical establishments readily accommodate such arrangements.

Another strategy that will help you generate some extra cash is eliminating some of the "extras" that you really do not need. For example, your home phone service is probably charging you for some extra services such as caller identification, call waiting, etc. If you cancel these options, you are likely save at least twenty percent off your monthly bill. Also, get rid of the unnecessary television cable and you can save at least fifty dollars a month. I am sure that you can think of many more "leisurely" services that you can certainly eliminate and have extra dollars.

These money saving techniques helped me take control of our finances. Once I was organized, I was on my way to securing a good line of credit, and to my surprise some creditors even wrote off our medical accounts!

Even through this tough situation, make time to talk to your ill spouse or family member. It is important that you try to lead a normal life as much as possible. Tony and I had very different daily schedules, but we always had our evening meal together. This was the time to catch up, just talk about the daily occurrences, and a time to nourish our relationship. We even made short-term goals! Yes, we made plans for a future…

Tony's cancer has been in remission for the last six years, and thanks be to God, we are almost done paying those old medical bills!

I still don't know why Tony was destined to suffer through this cancer ordeal. I may never know the answer to that question this side of heaven But we found a way to overcome the illness and as a result, matured as individuals. Our relationship is stronger than ever. Although we do not know why Tony had to fight this battle with cancer, it is enough to know that "the steps of the righteous are ordered by God."

What an Experience!
(Carol Remembers)

I vividly recall horrific the day my world shattered, my thoughts tired to escape in every direction as the doctor pronounced the word "Tumor". I kept hearing his words, "We found a brain tumor pressing on the and thus being the cause of the infamous headaches!" resonate in mind.

Once my brain clearly registered the word "Tumor!", the questions rampaged through my head. What? A tumor? It can't be! What are we going to do? My brain reeled with fear and confusion as I rushed out of the emergency room to gasp some air. In complete shock, my mind seemed to race at a one hundred miles an hour. I knew I had to calm down, but I could not! Uncontrollably, I cried out. After a few minutes, I regained enough control to return to the hospital. I went to Tony's room in search of his mom. We hugged each other. I remember just holding one another as tears rolled down our cheeks. Neither one of us knew what to say to comfort each other. We were beyond comfort. In fact, we were so busy being "beyond comfort" that it was several moments before we (finally) remembered that we had walked out on Tony, leaving him alone with the doctor!

Slowly but surely we walked back to find him. Like always he comforted us by saying, "Either way with God I don't lose." When the doctor talked to me, I felt a sense of peace. Somehow I knew that everything was going to be alright! Little did I know that, through trials and tribulations, both our faith and our family bonds would become stronger.

As the days went by, Tony had surgery, radiation treatments and rehabilitation therapy. Eight months later, just when we thought the long recovery process was over, the tumor regenerated with full strength.

The doctor said, "Hmmm…we're looking at another surgery." The tug of war between my brain and my heart started all over again. Against all odds, I said, "No more! There's got to be a better option!"

However, I knew that, as I took time to consider other alternatives, the malignant tumor world be creeping along and gaining more and more territory in my husband's brain. Without insurance, and with nothing other than faith and only hope on our side, we went to Herman Hospital in Houston. They turned us away because of the high cost of the treatments and the devastating nature of this particular cancer prognosis. Tony and I went home with such a sense of helplessness and disillusionment that I cannot even begin to find words to describe it.

Like it or not, life went on. I went back to my teaching job. After a few days, a friend brought me an article on a new brain procedure being performed at the M. D. Anderson Clark Cancer Clinic. I took the article home and it lay on my coffee table for days. As amazing as it may seem, I could not bring myself to read the article. Reading that article could get my hopes up; and if Tony were not accepted at that hospital, he and I would have to go through another immense disappointment. I just couldn't bear to see him discouraged a second time!

Nonetheless, by the end of that week, I armed myself with courage and read the article. The article reported that a Dr. Sawaya, the head of the neurosurgeon clinic, was utilizing a new laser surgery to remove brain tumors. Apparently this surgery was only being performed in two places in the world: the renowned Mayo Clinic and at M. D. Anderson hospital. A few weeks earlier, I had written to M.D. Anderson with respect to our dilemma, asking them to consider treating my husband.

As incredible as this may seem, that same evening at about 7:30 p. m. the phone rang. At first I hesitated to answer the call. I had grown tired of arguing with collection agencies asking for more money to cover medical expenses. Frankly, I just wasn't up to another fight. But something made me answer the phone. Although unwilling, I picked up the receiver and answered the call.

"Hello?"

"Good evening, this is Doctor Sawaya from M.D. Anderson Hospital. I urgently need to speak with Reverend Tony Perez," he requested.

My mind reeled with the shock of what I had just heard. My heart belied what my ears had heard.

"Excuse me. Who is this?" I replied.

"Dr. Sawaya, Are you Tony's wife?" the voice on the other end questioned.

I could hardly speak. I suppose he suspected this was the case, since he patiently waited for my response.

"Yes, sir, this is his wife Carol," I exclaimed.

I vividly recall the next part of the conversation. I had to advise him that Tony was not home at that time.

"Where is Tony? It is urgent that I speak to him."

"Dr. Sawaya, I know you're not going to believe it." I had to pause here, because even I couldn't believe what I was about to tell him. "He's, ahhh, out jogging, sir."

Now it was Dr. Sawaya's turn to pause and gather his thoughts!

He was out jogging! Can you imagine a guy with a death sentence hanging over his head going out and exercising? Well, that was Tony. He was full of vibrant energy and was deliberately spending every minute of his daily run in prayer and meditation.

Dr. Sawaya cleared his throat and said in his fatherly voice, "I understand that you have been through an ordeal. I have reviewed his scans and he is a good candidate for surgery and treatment. Do not do anything anymore. Stay put! Within a couple of weeks, I will get everything ready and then you all can come to meet the staff and we'll take care of surgery preparations."

You can only imagine what followed. For the very first time, someone understood what we were going through! Tears of joy and gratefulness started to fill my eyes. In that very moment, I realized that God made a way where there seemed to be no way!

It would be unrealistic (not to mention untrue) to pretend that, after Dr. Sawaya's call, everything was a breeze. Tony did have a successful surgery performed by very caring specialized doctors and nurses. However, the treatments were severely aggressive and they really tried our patience. I had to learn to cook bland meals free of processed ingredients for each of Tony's three meals a day. I had to wake up endless times in the middle of the night to nurse him. I was the one who had to pay the bills that could be paid and handle the calls from the collection agency for the ones that couldn't. Not only that, but I had to teach 26 little ones at school every day.

If it wouldn't have been for the incredible love and support of caring family and friends that were always ready to step in and help with finances, home cooked meals and cleaning my house, I would not have been able to give Tony the support and attention that he needed. The only concern that Tony voiced was his desire in knowing that I was still fulfilling life.

One day Tony said,

"Carol, I have been thinking. I believe you should go back to school and get your master's degree."

I immediately answered, "No way! I can't even handle what I have on my plate now! And you think I need more?"

"Yes, your desire has always been to get your master's. You need to get out of the house and do what you like!"

Once Tony progressed to a health optimal level, I did go back to college! Where did the money and energy come from? Again, God provided. You won't believe it, but the school district that employed me, offered a scholarship program in which I was accepted. To my amazement, I still performed all of my duties and always made time to sit with Tony to have our evening meal.

Through this experience, the relationship Tony and I shared has become deeper and better. We became the best of friends, and we learned to live each day as if it was the last! Today, Tony's tumor has been in remission for the last six years.

During the last doctor's visit, his oncologist said,

"Tony you are surely going to die of old age! Go live your life!"

And that's just what Tony is doing…

APPENDIX

MEETING JESUS

- The bible says God loves you so much He offers you eternal life once your life on this earth is through: "For God so loved the world that He gave His only Son, that whosoever believes in Him should not perish, but have everlasting life through Jesus Christ our Lord." John 3:16

- "For the wages of sin is death, but the gift of God is eternal life through Jesus Christ our Lord". Romans 6:23

The Bible says everyone has sinned, and sin separates you from God:

- "As it is written, there is none righteous, no, not one." Romans 3:10

- "For all have sinned and come short of the glory of God." Romans 3:23

The Bible tells of God's solution to the problem of your sin:

- "Christ died for our sins according to the scriptures; and He was buried and He rose again the third day according to the scriptures." I Corinthians 15:3,4

- Jesus said, "I am the way, the truth, and the life: no man comes to the Father (God) but by Me." John 14:6

The Bible says you can be saved!

- Behold I stand at the door and knock, and if any man hears My voice and opens the door, I will come in to him." Revelation 3:20

- "For whoever calls upon the name of the Lord shall be saved." Romans 10:13

- "If you confess with your mouth the Lord Jesus, and believe in your heart that God raised Him from the dead, you will be saved." Romans 10:9

The Bible says you are saved by faith:

- For by grace are you saved through faith—not of yourselves: it is the gift of God, not of works, lest any man should boast." Ephesians 2:8,9

So what should you do if you want to meet Jesus?

- Admit to God that you are a sinner.

- Tell Him you are sorry for your sins.

- Believe that Jesus has forgiven you completely and taken the punishment for your past, present and future sins.

- Accept Jesus as your personal Savior and friend.

- Invite Jesus to be the Lord of your life.

- Find a Bible-believing church and tell someone there about your decision to follow Jesus!

Just tell him in your own words or pray this prayer:
"Lord Jesus, I know that I am a sinner. I believe you died in my place to take away the punishment for my sins. I want you to be the Lord of my life. Please come into my heart so that I may follow you. Thank you for loving me so much. In Jesus' name I pray AMEN."

To contact Tony Peres for speaking engagements, please e-mail him at tonyncarol@aol.com, or write him at: 1710 E. 24th St., Mission, Texas 78574.

0-595-32303-0

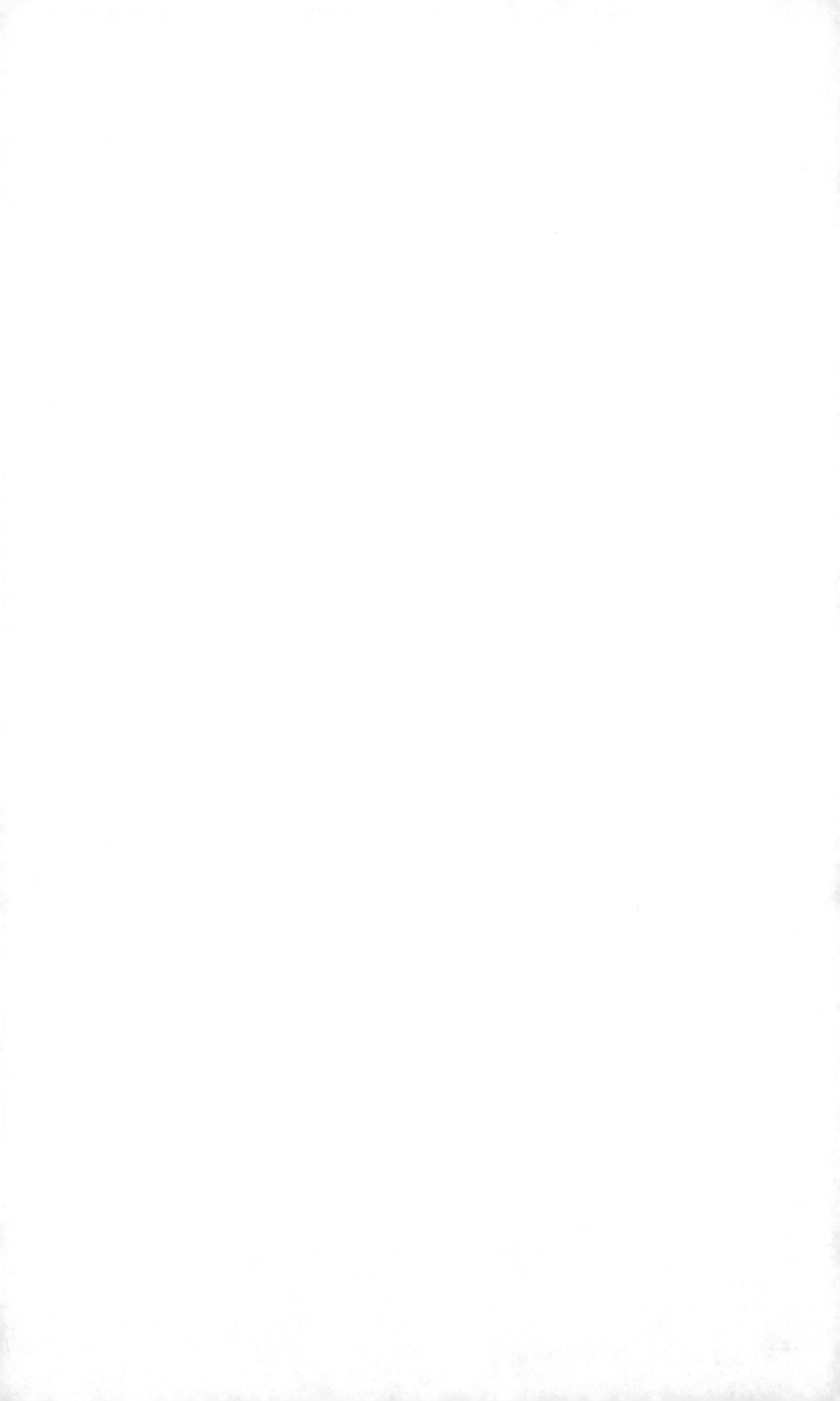

www.ingramcontent.com/pod-product-compliance
Lightning Source LLC
Chambersburg PA
CBHW031331290526
45784CB00014B/2551